Reconnecting With Your Inner Caveman

By Mick Reade

©2012

This is a story, over 2 million years in the making, about how to achieve optimum health through healthy diet and exercise, based on scientific evidence and archaeological research.

Human evolution achieved the peak of health about 10,000 years ago, discover how to restore your health and vitality as a modern hunter-gatherer, and reconnect with your "inner caveman"!

Index

Chapter One

Introduction - The Background of Our Background

If the artistic renderings of Paleolithic humans are any indication, our early ancestors weren't much to look at, by today's standards. Their low foreheads were accented by heavy brows, their noses were broad and somewhat flat, their jaws were prominent, and they were quite hairy. Modern analysts insist that this depiction has no basis, and that early representatives of our species were actually not much different in appearance from what we look like now. And yet the illustrations persist. Whatever the case, however they looked we know they had their health. They had to—life was rough in those days.

While many people today tend to think of Paleolithic man as a sort of every-man-for-himself lone wolf-type character, there actually was a communal society of sorts. People tended to live together in small bands, or tribes, where they could apportion the work, share the resources, and watch each other's backs. Their everyday tasks were basic: find food, move to a new location, find food, build shelter, find food, make tools and clothing, find food, look after the kids, find food, stay alive. They lived in the moment, never having to worry about finding and holding employment; it was their job to bring home the bacon—literally—and they could never even think about taking a sick day. The future was abstract, so why think about it? Life was all about the here and now—very simple, relatively low-maintenance, highly stressful at times, and generally quite happy.

Paleolithic man lived by the laws of nature. When the sun rose, so did he. He would breakfast on whatever food had been acquired on the previous day, and then set out to find sustenance for the rest of that day, and perhaps the next, if nature cooperated. His method of procuring food was through the process of hunting, gathering, and fishing. The menu depended on the geographic location, as well as the season.

What was important for all of our ancestors, whatever their location, was getting enough food to supply the necessary protein, fats, and calories to give them the energy they needed to sustain them in their search for more food. Where vegetation was plentiful, they ate their fill of fruits, greens, roots, tubers, stalks, and other plant food. This was probably experimental for a while, as some plants were toxic and would make them sick–or kill them. Doubtless our large-brained ancestors were quick studies who learned really fast which plants to look for, and which to avoid.

In fact, you may be surprised to learn that in contrast to the common view that our ancestors were primitive, unintelligent (some may say stupid) humans that just made grunting noises and bashed things, they were actually far more intelligent than we thought. Matt Ridley, who wrote *The Agile Gene*, reported that the average human brain size in 50,000 B.C. was 1,567cc for males and 1,468cc for females. Today that figure is 1,248cc for males and 1,210 for females… our brain size has actually been shrinking!

Considering the amount of energy required to do the stalking, running, jumping, and climbing our relatives had to do when they were on the hunt for food, it would have taken a rather substantial amount of plant food to provide it, so naturally they needed something more. Meat provided protein, fat, and calories to keep them going, so game had to be a large part of their diet. Small animals were pretty easy; throw a stone, use a club or a spear, and there's the meal.

While the small animals were likely a mainstay of their diet, cave paintings show that large animals such as bison, mammoths, and wild goats also played a role in the Paleolithic food plan. Many of these animals were not so easy to hunt; they had strength and speed that humans didn't have. Not only that, predatory animals like saber-tooth tigers and cave bears were likely to turn around and make a meal of their pursuers. Paleo man had to have an eat-or-be-eaten attitude to make it from one day to the next.

When the time came to prepare the food, great care was taken to avoid waste of any kind. For Paleo-man, nourishment was essential, so it is unlikely that there were any picky eaters in the band. Any part of the catch that was edible was part of the diet— muscle, organs, even the bone marrow.

Before fire became widely used for cooking, many of our ancient ancestors undoubtedly ate their game raw, but eventually they learned how to roast meat on a spit, or perhaps in a container with liquid to make a form of stews or soups. When the edible portions of the game were gone, the bones and antlers were used to make tools, and the skins were prepared for clothing and shelter.

The women in the band would usually take on the role of gatherers, although anthropologists generally believe they may have assisted in hunting smaller animals or helping to drive the larger ones off of cliffs. To accompany the meat course of the meal, they would find berries and other fruits, different vegetables as they were available, roots and tubers, seeds and nuts, and birds' eggs. Obviously, processed foods and sugar were never an option during this era; if there were such a thing as a sweet tooth back then, it had to be satisfied with the natural sweetness in fruits, or possibly with honey. More than likely, though, sweet cravings were never an issue.

The goal of Paleo-man was to stay satisfied, so most of his effort was devoted to finding the food, then doing whatever it took to get it back to the group. This could involve walking great distances over rough terrain to find prey; climbing trees, rocks or hills to survey the landscape; ducking under low branches; running in pursuit of alarmed quarry; and ultimately lifting the game and carrying it back to camp. To complicate matters even more, he always had to fight the elements and watch out for predators. It was a hard job, this day-to-day survival.

Meanwhile, Paleo-woman was busy augmenting her food-gathering chores by collecting wood and water, repairing tools, maintaining the shelter, butchering meat and preparing food, and caring for children (which included carrying each child until he or she was about four years old). Besides walking for many miles, these tasks required an extensive amount of lifting and carrying, bending, stretching, climbing, and digging. It was quite a workout, by any standards.

Imagine the impact that this lifestyle must have had on the health and fitness of our ancestors. Their diet was all-natural, low-carb, high protein, and full of essential vitamins and minerals they didn't even know they needed! They never had to set aside time to exercise because their daily activities represented what we would call interval training in our time.

Paleo men and women naturally had remarkable physical stamina, strength, agility, and resilience. In fact they most closely resembled a modern day Olympic decathlete - strong, lean, athletic, flexible, and capable of adapting quickly to whatever threats and challenges the surrounding environment would throw at them. Their cardiovascular systems were never compromised by a sedentary lifestyle or a diet that loaded their veins with sludge. They balanced the amount of work they did with periods of rest, so they never suffered from sleep deprivation. Moreover, their time outdoors ensured a sturdy skeletal system as they absorbed vitamin D from a natural source—the Sun.

Of course, with evolution, change was inevitable. Society evolved. Cultures evolved. Technology evolved. Man evolved—intellectually, anyway. Ironically, man's genetic makeup did not evolve. After all, our species had spent around two million years as hunter gatherers eating the fruits of our labors; we couldn't evolve overnight just to accommodate the new foods we were introducing to our systems. Our constitutions remained basically the same as they were when we were immensely active hunter-gatherers.

Regrettably, as we allowed ourselves to embrace the new shortcuts and conveniences that progress conferred on us, our bodies began to get soft, fragile, and sickly. The agricultural and industrial revolutions removed the need for us to provide for all our own requirements; now our role in society was limited to whatever specialty we could contribute, and, in turn, we depended on the work of others to supply us with our daily essentials like food, shelter, and clothing. We started keeping regular hours, and we changed our lifestyle.

Instead of eating a variety of healthy foods, we began to depend on processed foods that were convenient, tasty, and detrimental to our health. Rather than regularly engaging in a variety of physical challenges, we became content to just sit around; after all, we were no longer in a struggle to survive—why waste energy unnecessarily?

There are those who would argue that, just because Paleolithic man seemed to be a perfect physical specimen and didn't show signs of the maladies that plague us in our modern times—coronary disease, obesity, hypertension, diabetes, arthritis, among others—there's no evidence that these conditions wouldn't have developed if their life-spans had been longer. Well, actually, there is evidence: there are still some hunter-gatherer societies existing today, although not many. These modern-day hunter gatherers continue to be untouched by progress and maintain the same type of "uncivilized" lifestyle as our predecessors. Consequently, they are slim, strong, and fit. If there is any occurrence of modern maladies among them, it is extremely uncommon.

Chapter 2

The Agricultural Revolution - Where It All Started To Go Horribly Wrong

In the years 8000-5000 BC, the hunter-gatherer lifestyle was virtually obliterated by a revolution—the very first agricultural revolution, also called the Neolithic Revolution. Note the extremeness of the word Revolution. We don't call it a transition, we don't call it a phase, we don't call it a shift. A revolution, by definition, tends to take the status quo and turn it upside-down. It's the best word for describing the changes that took place when the Paleolithic hunter-gatherers decided to change their nomadic habits that had spanned two million years, settle down, and become farmers. Instead of walking all over the lands to find food, they chose instead to grow plants and domesticate animals.

There is evidence to support this fact in archaeological explorations that have uncovered large caches of seeds—too large to have been only for human consumption. Many different theories attempt to explain why this transition may have happened; they run the gamut from changes in climate to rapidly growing population requirements to desires to show displays of power. Climate change, a buzz word of recent years and hotly debated, is a common theme throughout the ages, particularly through the Paleolithic Era when several Ice Ages covered the Earth for extended periods, and then receded (scientists refer to Ice Ages as "glaciation", and the periods in between as "interglacial periods").

It was around this time that the last Ice Age began to recede, and the time since then right up to the current day is an interglacial period. It's believed that many of the large animals of the Ice Age such as woolly mammoths, woolly rhinos, glyptodonts, cave bears, and other similar animals perfectly adapted to the cold were driven to extinction by a combination of the changing weather conditions, as well as being hunted for food by man.

The point is, something seems to have changed people's motivations, and it's possible that the changing weather also forced a change in the food source, as the previously plentiful supply increasingly became hard to come by. While it wasn't exactly a spontaneous linear shift across the planet, there is documented archaeological evidence of the same types of conversions occurring independently in six distinct areas throughout the world at some point during this period.

The Neolithic Revolution signaled the end of the small, rootless bands of hunter-gatherers. They transformed themselves into societies that built and settled communities, adopted food-crop specializations, and developed techniques and strategies to grow and harvest an actual surplus of food. While there was still some work involved in growing and harvesting crops and domesticating animals, the amount of daily physical effort didn't approach the level of the hunter-gatherer lifestyle.

The new Neolithic agrarian values encouraged a more sedentary lifestyle, at the same time profoundly altering the natural environment. The sparse, temporary camps of the Paleolithic societies became densely populated settlements which required the clearing of forests, the re-direction of water sources, and the construction of permanent buildings to house people and store crops.

Whereas Paleolithic children were nourished on mother's milk, and only until they were weaned, Neolithic man began to appreciate the value of animals like cows and goats as sources of milk that people of all ages could drink. Moreover, they found that domesticated animals could also provide a source of protein that could be continuously replenished by breeding the animals. As a bonus, animals also provided hides, wool, and fertilizer, and they could be trained to work for man—plowing fields, towing supplies, and, in the case of dogs, helping to control other animals. The earliest domesticated animals included sheep and pigs, in addition to the dogs, cows, and goats.

As society continued to evolve, labor became diversified, a trading system was developed, and man could relax a little more since he didn't have to take care of every little necessity himself. He was on the fast road to becoming soft—and the new diet he began to adopt represented the maximum speed limit.

The first sign of trouble was the selective propagation of cereal grasses—emmer, einkorn, and barley were the first to be grown successfully. Grains had been a problem for Paleo man. For one thing, the early versions were small; they yielded paltry quantities; and they had to be milled to make them edible; so they were really more trouble than they were worth, even if they weren't toxic. That's the other problem with grains—in their uncooked state they contain toxins, which we would call anti-nutrients these days.

Eventually millet, rice, wheat, corn, and beans were added to the human diet, and later rye, oats, and sorghum. Obviously, some of these foods were not available everywhere—climate and geography played a big part in the availability of grains in certain locales.

When we realize that the digestive system of the hunter-gatherer remained virtually unchallenged by any change in diet at all for a span of two million years, it puts the ten thousand years, or 500 generations, of "modern" diet into a new perspective. Evolution doesn't occur overnight, and ten thousand years is relatively overnight when we compare it to two million years. As primates, our digestive systems do not have the means of breaking down the fiber in grains. In fact, the cell walls of grains are nearly entirely unaffected by the GI processes, and they can pass through the digestive system completely intact. We need to mill them to break down the cell walls to have access to the carbohydrate and protein calories in cereal grains, and we also need to cook them to reduce the effect of the toxins (note that the toxins are not always entirely eliminated) and make the starches more digestible.

Once cooking techniques were established, grains began to be perceived as a perpetual source of nutrition for man, thereby establishing themselves as a foundation of the Neolithic diet. As we learned more about agriculture, we developed strains with larger grains that could be more easily harvested, and the crops themselves became more abundant. This created a surplus, which in turn necessitated the creation of a system for food storage. Unfortunately, man's genetic makeup has not evolved to the degree that our diet has, and our digestive systems are incompatible with the "new" foods adopted by our Neolithic forbears.

While some people may have believed that these changes in diet and lifestyle were positive, there is evidence to suggest that any thoughts of health benefits were left along the wayside with the adoption of the new habits and diet. There was an obvious decline in the hardiness of men and women after this change in lifestyle. The average height of men and women in the Neolithic age actually decreased by about 15-20cm, and they stayed in that range until the twentieth century. This diminishment in height suggests that the quality of the new nutritional paradigm was substandard to the regimen that had been abandoned. This physical decline quite likely could have increased vulnerability to disease and shortened life expectancy.

You may be scratching your head in bewilderment right now, thinking, "But I eat grains with no problem. What's the big deal?" And, of course, cereal companies talk about the importance of cereal's fiber in the diet and claim that their products will keep us healthy. But don't forget that these products have had to be "fortified" with vitamins and minerals to compensate for the nutrients that have been lost in the process of the preparing them for human consumption. Since we can get vitamins, minerals, and fiber from so many other natural, unprocessed sources, it's basically pointless to get our calories from grains that can actually do more harm than good.

How, exactly, can grains in our diet be harmful to our health? It's true that most of us do have a certain degree of tolerance to grains, but just because we can eat them, and we seem to be able to digest them, doesn't mean they're providing us with the health benefits our bodies need to thrive. The evolutionary design of our digestive systems actually makes it impossible to digest the grains efficiently; it leaves their nutrients unavailable for proper absorption by the body. In fact, some of the components of grains (phytates) actually bind themselves to the minerals in the grains and actively prevent them from being assimilated, thereby counteracting their potential benefits.

Our bodies have been genetically programmed to digest the *macronutrients* in our foods: the proteins, carbohydrates, and fats. *Micronutrients* are also essential to our bodies, but in smaller quantities. There is also another component in some foods, including grains, known as *antinutrients*. These elements actually have a toxic effect on the body. Phytates are just one group of components in grain that are categorized as antinutrients. Others are lectins and glutens. These substances are capable of causing all kinds of pandemonium to our bodily processes.

Take lectins, for instance. These little suckers are actually in ALL foods we consume. Some are your enemies, some are your friends, and some are like Switzerland (neutral). Think of a lectin as a protein containing a key that fits a certain type of lock. This lock is a specific type of carbohydrate. All life forms, plant and animal, insect and fungus have cell membranes that contain carbohydrates that sit within and project from the membrane. If a lectin with the right key comes in contact with one of these 'locks' on the gut wall or artery or gland or organ it 'opens the lock'.

They tend to attach themselves to our intestinal lining, impeding the absorption of nutrients and significantly reducing the number of healthy bacteria in our guts. Without these important digestive functions, stomach and intestinal problems will occur. Researchers have also discovered that lectins actually inhibit the body's processes to repair the GI tract, which creates the potential for material from the digestive system to leak into the bloodstream. When this happens, our immune system is challenged, and autoimmune disorders can be the result.

Lectin consumption also seems to be connected to a condition known as leptin resistance. Leptin is the hormone that communicates to our brain our need to consume food for energy—or not. If our brain doesn't get the right signals at the right time, we could find ourselves overeating, and worse. A resistance to leptin can cause problems such as elevated blood pressure, high insulin levels, undesirable cholesterol readings, and surplus body fat in the waist area, even if obesity isn't a factor. This increases the risk for heart disease, stroke, and diabetes. Furthermore, lectins can increase our chances of viral illnesses, as some viruses actually use lectins as agents for attaching themselves to host cells during infection.

Lectins can be inactivated by specific carbohydrates (technically known as mono and oligosaccarides) which can bind the 'key' and prevent the protein from attaching to the carbohydrate 'lock' within the cell membrane. Glucosamine is specific for wheat lectin and it is this specificity that may protect the gut and cartilage from cell inflammation and destruction in wheat (or gluten) responsive arthritis.

While various foods and supplements may inactivate some of these toxic lectins it is impossible for such substances to protect the body from them completely. The safest way is to avoid known toxic lectins. Common foods with known toxic lectins include all soy and wheat products, including oils from these substances, as well as dairy (particularly from grain-fed cows).

Another antinutrient, gluten, may have a more familiar ring to most people. It's received a good deal of attention in the media because gluten sensitivity poses a serious problem to a wide spectrum of people. As a matter of fact, researchers have come to the conclusion that as many as 85% of us have some kind of gluten intolerance or sensitivity (although many don't necessarily realize it). For those people, the body sees gluten as a threat, like a virus, and the immune defenses go to work to fight against the danger. In the process, surrounding tissue receives collateral damage, which creates an inflammatory response, which leads to many other problems.

At its worst, gluten sensitivity could be manifested in the form of Celiac Disease, which is well known to cause extreme misery in the form of severe abdominal pain and diarrhea. But the difficulties don't stop there; by continuing to consume such gluten-loaded foods as bread, pasta, cookies and other pastries, and pizza, sufferers are causing damage to the lining of the small intestine, making the absorption of some nutrients impossible. The vitamin deficiencies that result can affect the brain, bones, nervous system, liver, and other vital organs.

Even if Celiac disease is not the diagnosis, gluten-sensitive people can experience acid reflux, fatigue, low energy, autoimmune disorders, fibromyalgia, muscle and joint pain, skin rashes, and some problems with co-ordination. Some sufferers have even reported cognitive dysfunction and numbness in the extremities.

Phytates, while not as familiar a term as gluten, are antinutrients that can bind themselves to important minerals like calcium, magnesium, and zinc, and make them difficult or impossible for the cells to absorb. Even the minerals in the so-called fortified breads and cereals are rendered unusable by the phytates present in the very same grains. Nursing mothers should be especially careful about their consumption of foods containing phytates, as the mineral shortages they cause can delay development in their infants.

Since the whole point of eating (originally, before it became recreational) is to acquire calories to provide energy so that we can accomplish daily tasks, it's much better to avoid the calories in grains and opt for the Paleo recommendations of lean meats, seafood, vegetables, and fruits. These foods provide a much better way of getting fiber, B vitamins and minerals. In fact, according to the book *The Paleo Diet* by Dr. Loren Cordain, "an average 1,000 calorie serving of mixed vegetables contains 19 times more folate, five times more vitamin B-6, six times more vitamin B-2 and two times more vitamin B-1 than a comparable serving of eight mixed whole grains." If we added up all the calories we would consume if we were to get the same amount of nutrients only from grains, the resulting effect on our bodies wouldn't be healthy— or pretty.

Chapter 3

Killing Me Sweetly

Just when our Paleolithic genetics had begun to think our bodies had been assaulted with as much alien fodder as we could tolerate, sugar entered the picture. At first, it seemed pretty innocuous, as indigenous people would cut sugar cane and chew on it for its sweetness. But eventually—actually, only within the past 200 years—we found a way to refine it, and refined sugar began to actually replace our healthy unrefined carbohydrates.

Sugar can be quite an addictive substance for many of us, and I'm sure you've most likely heard the term "sweet tooth" thrown around. Before we learned how to refine sugar, this sweet tooth came in very handy for hunter-gatherers. Man discovered (largely by trial-and-error to begin with) that many of the edible plants in nature that were not poisonous to us tended to be sweet, leading us to the obvious conclusion that, in general, if it was sweet it's ok to eat. This was useful for avoiding a horrible death by poison and led to berries and fruits becoming a great food staple, however the past 200 years has seen us take this "if it's sweet, it's good to eat" theory to the extreme with catastrophic results.

We've all heard the term "empty calories" applied to sugar, but that term seems almost innocent in light of the way sugar acts once it gets into our system. Health wise, sugar really has nothing going for it—no protein, no minerals, no vitamins, not even any fiber. Since refined sugars have no nutrient value of their own, they steal the minerals and vitamins that the body has taken in from other foods. The sugar manipulates these nutrients to assist in its own metabolism into the system.

Now, with fewer of these nutrients available for normal systemic processes, cholesterol and fatty acid cannot be properly metabolized, which causes triglyceride and cholesterol levels to rise. In addition, as insulin is released, the body's blood-sugar balance is thrown out of kilter, and more fatty acid is stored around organs and in areas just beneath the skin, which leads to obesity. All of these factors create a greater risk for cardiovascular disease.

People who crave sugar look for that short burst, or "rush" of energy, but when that burst fizzles out, we're often left feeling more sluggish than we were in the first place, a condition that's come to be known as a "sugar crash". The rush is attributed to the rapid rise in blood glucose after consuming a large quantity of sugar or other processed carbohydrates. Our bodies react to this increase by secreting the hormone insulin, which then stimulates the tissues into either rapidly using the glucose for energy production or storing it as glycogen. Once it's been used or stored, blood glucose falls, and we "crash."

There's more to say about insulin; it was one of the first hormones to evolve in man and other living things, and at the time it was a great necessity. It acts as an agent for storing nutrients that aren't immediately required by our bodies. Because of the inconsistency of the food supply, our Paleolithic ancestors very likely had to deal with alternating periods of feast and famine. In order to survive during times when food was scarce, the stored nutrients were essential to sustain them until the next meal. At that point in our development as a species, it was a very efficient means of dealing with our environment.

Ten thousand years later, researchers believe insulin has come to a point where it's being overworked in our modern bodies. Our ancestors' bodies didn't put too many demands on insulin because they had no access to refined sugars, and very few opportunities to take in any other form of sugar or carbohydrates. After all, even the healthier complex carbohydrates like fruits and vegetables were only available in the summer and fall. In our modern times, we have constant access to all kinds of sugars and refined carbohydrates, and we don't have to work very hard to get them. So, of course there will be surplus for most of us.

When we over-indulge on sugar, our pancreas—mindful of its intrinsic duty—goes into action secreting insulin to get that extra glucose into storage, only there's no room for it because the liver and muscle cells are already full of glycogen. They have no choice other than to develop a resistance to the commands of insulin. They begin to reduce the number and proficiency of the insulin receptors on their surface and make it even more difficult for the glucose to get into the cells.

When the pancreas detects that the toxic glucose is still hanging around in the bloodstream, it sends out more insulin, creating even more resistance, which creates excess insulin, which creates even more toxicity! This is a critical problem, and as a solution, our bodies have developed a system to direct the extra glucose to be stored in fat cells.

Remember, this process didn't start out as a problem with too much fat—it started out as a problem with too much sugar! In fact, sugar is far more likely than fat to cause obesity in most people. Especially problematic is the popularity of juices and carbonated drinks containing sugar and/or high-fructose corn syrup. People, especially teens and adolescents, tend to consume these beverages thoughtlessly, adding more total calories to their daily intake without actually accounting for them. Then they get an ugly surprise the next time they step on a scale.

Besides adding to our fat stores, insulin resistance makes building and maintaining our muscles more difficult by preventing important amino acids from entering the muscle cells. If that weren't enough, we experience a drop in energy, and we actually begin to crave more of the carbohydrates that are creating all of these problems in the first place. We're also likely to feel fatigued, making it less likely that we'll exercise those extra calories away.

The list continues of the potential problems that sugar poses for our health—problems that worsen over time if we don't change our habits. For one thing, sugar takes a toll on the body's immune system. Because it's absorbed more rapidly than healthy complex carbohydrates, sugar goes to work immediately to raise the body's insulin levels. Then a domino effect begins: when the insulin level rises, growth hormones are not released as readily, and the immune system is compromised. In fact, just one tablespoon of sugar can degrade the body's immune system for as long as six hours. A weakened immune system means a greater susceptibility to disease, so people who consume sugar in excessive quantities may find that they experience frequent illness.

In addition to the problems already mentioned, habitual sugar consumption is also recognized as a primary offender in such conditions as type 2 diabetes, osteoporosis, kidney, liver, and heart disease, depression and mood swings, some nervous disorders, gallstones, and arthritis. Even cancer can be affected by sugar, since cancer cells thrive and tumors grow when they're bolstered by sugar. And we mustn't forget the detrimental effect sugar has on our teeth and gums—we've been hearing about that since childhood.

To be fair, sugar isn't the only culprit when it comes to wreaking havoc with our bodies. All carbohydrates—bread, cereals, potatoes, pasta, rice, etc.—are actually converted to glucose after they're eaten. And we already know what happens when we have too much glucose in our blood stream. And because a surplus of glucose can't be removed from the bloodstream quickly enough (don't blame the poor pancreas, it's really, really trying), it tends to make our circulatory systems more sluggish, binding with proteins to create more harmful substances that contribute to inflammation.

At this point, the pancreas has become worn out and can't produce the insulin any more. Now, if we're genetically predisposed (as many of us are, unfortunately), we find that we have acquired insulin-dependent Type-2 diabetes, and now we have to inject the insulin into our bodies. All this because of sugar and processed carbohydrates!

For most of us, unless we get consistent vigorous exercise, consuming more than 300 grams of carbohydrates a day is an assault on our bodies of excessive insulin, resulting in excessive storage of fat. Each time our bodies respond to this assault, the pancreas, the adrenal system, and the immune system have to bear the burden, and over time a new wrinkle is added—our bodies begin to feel the signs of *chronic* inflammation, and they launch into repair mode. This involves the production of free radicals in response to the inflammation.

Unfortunately, free radicals don't confine themselves to the problem areas—they also cause destruction in healthy cells and DNA. As long as our bodies are busy fighting chronic inflammation, our immune system is less able to deal with potential bacterial, viral, and fungus infections. All these things could have been avoided if we had only avoided the foods that our ancient ancestors avoided.

Now let's look at another food that was not consumed by our ancestors: dairy. Obviously, cheese was not an item that could be foraged in the wilderness, butter didn't grow on trees, and milk was only for children up to about four years old, when they were weaned from mother's milk. After that age, milk was never a part of Paleo man's diet.

When the Agricultural Revolution introduced the milk of cows and goats into the diet of humans past the age of four, we began to discover the discomfort of milk allergy and lactose intolerance. Lactose is yet another form of sugar. This sugar takes a specific enzyme, lactase, for digestion, and adults tend to stop producing as much lactase in their intestines as they mature from childhood. This is when symptoms can develop. The lining of the small intestine becomes inflamed, and the abdomen is clobbered by cramps in response to the swelling and irritation. Symptoms of lactose intolerance can range anywhere from gas, bloating, and pain, to diarrhea, nausea, and vomiting.

An allergy to milk can produce similar symptoms, but the reaction is specifically tied to a hypersensitivity to whey and/or casein, which are the specific proteins found in dairy. People with an allergy to dairy products have immune systems that identify these proteins as harmful, and they attempt to defend the body by creating antibodies against them. The antibodies produce histamines, but the histamines produce inflammation, swelling, and the symptoms described above. These symptoms can begin just a few minutes after drinking milk, or they can take up to two hours to appear. Sometimes it's the things we love that hurt us the most.

Chapter 4

Good Fat, Bad Fat... And Why Cholesterol Isn't Our Biggest Enemy

Nutrition experts are everywhere: online, in bookstores and libraries, on television and radio, and on street corners. They all have valuable information to impart about good fat, bad fat, and cholesterol. And it's all very confusing. Our Paleolithic ancestors, on the other hand, never had to give fat and cholesterol a second thought. They certainly never took any pills to try to keep their weight, blood pressure, and cholesterol under control.

Let's face it—Paleo man most likely ate a good amount of fat, by today's standards, to go along with his consumption of lean meat. After all, research has shown that he seemed to have enjoyed high-fat delicacies like organ meat and bone marrow. For Paleo man, who needed all the energy and warmth he could get, fat was a friend, not a foe.

To confuse the issue of fat in our time even more, there are different types of fats. Some of them are labeled good fats, and some are considered bad fats. What we need to remember, though, is that just about all natural sources of fat are actually a combination of several types of fat, and food can have both good and bad fats in one source.

Let's start with saturated fats, the fats found in animal products and some tropical oils, like coconut oil and palm oil. For several decades, we've been warned against this "artery-clogging" fiend and the relationship between higher levels of fat consumption and heart disease. This idea was embraced by the scientific community upon the publication of the "Seven Countries Study" by Ancel Keys in the 1950s.

The fact is, the study actually involved twenty two countries, but Keys manipulated his information to fit his theory, rather than coming to a conclusion based on the entire body of evidence. In publishing and publicizing his study, he chose to leave out important details that didn't support his conjecture-based premise.

Today, although there is virtually no evidence to support his theories, people are still being warned against too much fat in their diet, and scientists continue to try to prove their point. Harvard researchers organized a comprehensive study of the subject that is still ongoing today, the Framingham study. The results of this study have not been formally published because the investigators could not prove there was a relationship between heart attack risk and the intake of saturated fat. In fact, several sources have acknowledged that they didn't discover any significant relationship between risk of heart attack, blood cholesterol levels, and intake of saturated fat.

One of the most recent studies was published in 1996, the Health Professional Follow-up study. This controlled study was comprehensive and well-funded, but the results were basically the same: there is no relationship between the consumption of saturated fat and blood cholesterol. Even though there might be a small effect on cholesterol, it increases *both* LDL and HDL levels, so it would be difficult to predict its effect on heart attack risk.

Looking back at our ancestors, data suggests that the intake of saturated fats could have been anywhere between 10% and 15% of the total energy obtained from food, which is a little beyond the 10% that's recommended by mainstream nutrition experts. Our genetic makeup was based on a diet that not only tolerated, but required a certain amount of saturated fat, and there has never been any evidence that our ancestors suffered from any degree of heart problems.

The truth is, saturated fats are an important part of a healthy diet. They make up half of the body's cell membrane structures, and they're instrumental in many of the body's functions, including absorption of calcium, immune efficiency, and the synthesis of fatty acids. Saturated fats are also a good source of fat soluble vitamins and cholesterol. (Don't cringe at the c-word. There's surprising information about that, too!)

Of course, although some diets will tell us to eat as much saturated fats as we want, it's important to avoid overindulging on anything. As with everything, saturated fat consumption should be balanced; protein from lean meats is still a key part of the Paleo diet, and basic lifestyle changes should be adopted to keep systemic inflammation under control. Exercising regularly (but not excessively), taking steps to lower stress levels, minimizing the consumption of alcohol, and refraining from smoking are all factors that will benefit heart health.

So now we know that there's another side to the saturated fat coin. But what, exactly makes a fat saturated or unsaturated? Generally, a fat that remains solid at room temperature is considered to be a saturated fat. The more solid, the more saturated, and the less easily digested. For example, compare the fat of bacon and chicken fat after they're cooked and cooled to room temperature. The bacon fat is relatively solid, and will not pour, while the chicken fat tends to be a little more liquid.

This indicates that the bacon fat is more saturated than the chicken fat. It's also a good illustration of the fact that, just because animal fat is called saturated, it doesn't indicate that the total fat is saturated. In fact, the chicken fat is actually about 70%, or more than half, *un*saturated. Fats from other meats vary, but in many cases, animal fats are less than half saturated. Even lard is 60% unsaturated, so calling animal fats saturated is a blatant case of misrepresentation.

Fats that are labeled "good" fats tend to lower cholesterol and triglyceride levels in the blood, thereby reducing the risk for heart disease. Unsaturated fats are generally characterized as good fats, and they're found in two forms: monounsaturated fats and polyunsaturated fats. These types of fats retain their liquid form at room temperature; the polyunsaturated fats, commonly referred to as PUFAs in the nutrition world, remain in liquid state liquid even when refrigerated.

While they're technically classified as good fats, PUFAs are actually a mixed bag. There are some in the Paleo community that recommend avoiding them completely, while others recognize that a small amount of PUFAs do belong in our diet and serve a definite purpose. For instance, they're a rich source of omega 3 and omega 6 fatty acids (which are whole different story in themselves).

We need PUFAs to build and maintain our cell membranes and protective nerve coverings. They also help to clear the body of newly formed cholesterol and lower the amount of fatty deposits in our arteries. They have a beneficial effect on our triglyceride and cholesterol levels, and they have anti-blood clotting properties, which have been shown to improve heart health by lowering blood pressure and reducing the risk of stroke, heart disease, and irregular heartbeat.

PUFAs also have anti-inflammatory properties that are effective in reducing risks for and alleviating symptoms of several non-circulatory diseases, including diabetes, lupus, rheumatoid arthritis, inflammatory bowel disease, eczema, and some cancers. They have even been shown to forestall mental decline. With all this nutritional value, why would anyone be opposed to PUFAs in the diet?

Actually, it's a matter of degree. As we have learned, our bodies manufacture and store some fat, and fat is one of the macronutrients essential to a healthy body. But we don't have the capacity to manufacture our own polyunsaturated fats, or PUFAs, so we need to get them from foods such as fish, nuts, leafy greens, algae, and seeds—especially flax seeds. Vegetable oils like corn, canola, sunflower, and safflower also contain PUFAs, but we have to be careful—if we take in more than small quantities of PUFAs in any form, we could be setting ourselves up for damage from free radicals.

That's the dark side of these particular "good" fats: they're chemically unstable and have a tendency to oxidize when heated, bringing out the free radicals. These are unstable atoms or groups of atoms in our bodies that attack other cells, and when they become excessive, they start to cause damage that results in everything from premature aging and wrinkles to liver damage, an impaired immune system, plaque accumulation in arteries, and even cancer. These risks can be avoided by ensuring that we have plenty of antioxidants and minerals in our diets to combat the oxidative properties of any foods we ingest, including polyunsaturated fats.

Moving right along, let's segue from the "questionable" fats (that term seems so much more appropriate than bad or good, in this case) to monounsaturated fats, which generally get the seal of approval as "good" fats from nutritionists and Paleo followers alike. Monounsaturated fats, or MUFAs (may as well be consistent), are found in avocados, olives, sesame seeds, pecans, hazelnuts, and some other fruits and vegetables. They have the ability to reduce levels of LDL (bad cholesterol) at the same time as they raise the HDL levels. They also lower triglycerides and support the body's growth and development by supplying essential vitamins.

As we would expect, MUFAs come with a load of health benefits, including lower risk of heart disease and stroke, a decreased risk of breast cancer, help in reducing belly fat and maintaining a healthy weight, and reduction of pain and stiffness levels in those who suffer from rheumatoid arthritis. There is also research showing that MUFAs are beneficial in controlling blood sugar and insulin concentrations.

So, we can confidently say that monounsaturated fats actually warrant the label "good fat" with no qualifications. Is there a fat that warrants the unqualified label "bad fat?" Well, yes and no. Trans-fats have been getting a good deal of negative attention in recent years, and most of them—the ones that don't occur naturally—are really bad.

Most trans-fats are man-made fats that have gone through a process that turns liquid oil into more solid forms of fat (think margarine and shortening). The process, called hydrogenation, involves taking hydrogen and injecting it into vegetable oils like corn oil, cottonseed oil, and others. The hydrogen then transforms the oils into solid form. Trans-fats are popular with some food companies because they provide a longer shelf life for baked goods, they add to the fry life of cooking oils, and they are less expensive than healthier oils. Some manufacturers believe they also enhance the flavor and texture of some foods.

Foods containing trans-fats aren't limited to margarine and shortening; many fried foods are absolutely wallowing in trans-fat. A typical serving of French fries, for example, has around 40 per cent trans-fat. Cookies, crackers and pastries are also carriers of trans-fats; an innocent cracker can have as much as 50 per cent of the villainous substance. Many other processed foods, such as cereals and frozen waffles, are also sources. Any suspicions can be confirmed by checking the label; food companies in many countries are now required to list trans-fats on nutrition labels. If there's any doubt, check the listing of ingredients for shortening, hydrogenated, or partially hydrogenated oil. If they're listed near the top of the list, that food item has a substantial percentage of trans-fats and should be avoided.

Trans-fats are bullies in the fat world; they actually displace healthy fats, such as omega-3 fatty acids, so that they're unable to provide their usual benefits to our bodies. We need to avoid trans-fats as much as possible because of the many detrimental effects they have on our bodies. Research shows that even small amounts of trans-fat in our diets put us at a higher risk for artery and heart disease by raising our LDL cholesterol levels. Harvard studies have shown that as many as 30,000 heart disease deaths a year could be related to trans-fat consumption.

In addition, trans-fats are known to promote insulin resistance (again?), aggravating conditions such as diabetes, hypertension, and obesity. They can also weaken the body's immune system, making us vulnerable to increased incidence of some types of cancer, and they can lower the efficiency of the liver. For men, trans-fats decrease levels of testosterone and increase the formation of abnormal sperm. In pregnant women, trans-fats can complicate pregnancy, increase the rate of low birth-weight babies, and produce substandard breast milk. Pretty bad stuff.

As previously indicated, however, there is a caveat to the bad trans fat; some trans fats are actually found in nature. They occur in the fat of ruminants (cows, bison, buffalo—animals that have partitioned stomachs and chew cuds) and in dairy fats. Grass-fed ruminants supply a higher percentage of these types of beneficial trans fats. There is an argument that the principal types of natural trans-fats from these sources can be converted to conjugated linoleic acid (CLA) in our bodies, which is not believed to retain the negative systemic effects of man-made trans fats, and is also believed to have properties that fight cancer.

Now, as if the issue weren't already complicated enough, we need to consider some sub-units of fats, omega 3 and omega 6 fatty acids. Since our bodies can't produce these substances, we call them "essential" fatty acids. Omega 6 acids are important to kidney function, skin, and a number of other things. These fatty acids can be found in grain-fed meat, corn, other grains, and those diabolical trans fats, so there must be a Paleo down side, and there is. When omega 6 fatty acids get out of control, they can trigger inflammation. To keep them from turning to the dark side, we need to balance them with omega 3s.

Omega 3 fatty acids are found in the foods that are rich in PUFOs, i.e., fish, algae, flax, and nuts. They aid circulation, fight against systemic inflammation, help maintain brain function, and reduce symptoms of such mental conditions as depression, anxiety, and ADHD.

The diet of our ancestors is thought to have been comprised of a ratio of 2:1 omega 6 acids to omega 3, although numbers on this subject vary. This is believed to be the optimal ratio. Current western diets are estimated to include a ratio of about 10:1, right up to 20:1 in some cases! That's a pretty serious imbalance, and it's a central factor in several types of chronic diseases, including cardiovascular disease, most inflammatory diseases, several psychological disturbances, and many cancers.

As long as we're discussing confusing issues regarding which foods are healthy and which are unhealthy, we need to turn our attention to the topic of cholesterol. When heart disease started to become a problem around the early part of the twentieth century, anxious doctors determined to find the cause. Initial tests conducted in the 1950s showed that there was evidently a connection between arterial fat deposits and lesions and premature death due to heart disease.

The presence of cholesterol in those fat deposits led researchers to the conclusion that cholesterol was a prime factor in the heart disease. This premise was supported by their previous association between heart disease and a family history of high cholesterol. Unfortunately, they ignored the fact that cholesterol is a vital part of our blood plasma and naturally needs to be present. They virtually declared war on heart disease and, with no real evidence, pointed to cholesterol as the enemy. In truth, 50 per cent of all people who experience a heart attack for the first time have a cholesterol profile in the normal range.

Cholesterol is a waxy, hard-working lipid (fat—again) found in our blood plasma and cells' membranes. Our bodies need cholesterol to insulate neurons, manufacture bile, metabolize fat soluble vitamins, build and maintain cellular walls, support learning and memory, and facilitate the synthesis of many of the body's hormones. To make sure our bodies have enough cholesterol to perform all these tasks, our liver produces about 1000 – 1400 milligrams of it every day. If we're getting some from the foods we eat, our livers take a little break and produce less. If we're not getting very much cholesterol from the foods we eat, the liver will produce more.

It was in the 1960s that cholesterol's reputation began to be significantly defamed, thanks again to Ancel Key's one-sided study. While his ideas hadn't immediately taken hold when his study was first published, he apparently did some lobbying to bring the scientific community and even the American Heart Association over to his way of thinking. He even managed to make it to the cover of *Time* magazine. As a result, advice began to proliferate to change our diet by cutting down on total fat, especially saturated fat and cholesterol from foods such as fatty meat, egg yolks, whole milk, and butter.

As it turned out, this advice was misguided, since our livers control our bodies' production of cholesterol according to what we get from our diet. If our bodies sense that we're not getting sufficient dietary cholesterol, our liver will manufacture it! For most of us, eating high-cholesterol foods has a negligible effect on our levels of blood cholesterol. Furthermore, even as we were warned against the dangers of cholesterol, it was also recommended that we incorporate more carbohydrates from grains as well as polyunsaturated seed oils into our diets (completely deviating from Paleo wisdom).

Dietary cholesterol and saturated fat were doomed to suffer from negative public opinion, especially after *Time* magazine showed support for the theory that cholesterol and heart disease were inextricably linked (in another very one-sided article). Again, some very important information was omitted from what the public saw: nearly every study suggests that it's only the *oxidized* LDL that creates the problems. The non-oxidized serum cholesterol is actually good for us, so our focus should be on the cause of cholesterol oxidation, which is free radicals, mostly from trans fats. The way to fight this oxidation problem is to avoid trans fats and to consume foods rich in *anti*-oxidants: fruits and vegetables, nuts, olive oil—the usual healthy Paleo fare.

The naysayers whose objective is to vilify cholesterol want us to focus on letters and numbers: LDL, HDL, and whatever number it is that measures the level in our blood. LDL, or low density lipoprotein, is considered the bad-guy of the cholesterol-forming team. (Think of L as Lousy). This component of cholesterol is used as a delivery system to carry the newly-manufactured cholesterol from the liver to the tissues. Our LDL levels tend to rise when we overindulge in *carbs and trans fats*, resulting in inflammation. Contrary to traditional belief, it doesn't have anything to do with our intake of saturated fat.

HDL is the acronym for high density lipoproteins, and this is the good-guy part of cholesterol. (Think of the H as Happy.) It's HDL's job to transfer cholesterol from body tissues to the liver, which eliminates it through the bile. HDL makes sure that, once the body is finished with it, excess cholesterol leaves the party. Consequently, if we eat plenty of foods to elevate our HDL level, our bodies will process cholesterol smoothly, and the bad cholesterol won't be able to do its dirty work.

If we have LDL levels less than 100, we're told that we're at low risk for heart disease, but if it gets up above 160, we're warned that we're in danger. If our LDL is above 190, we're in a lot of danger. Conversely, our HDL levels signal less risk for heart disease; that's why we want higher levels of the good cholesterol. A level of 60 and above means lower risk, and a level of 40 or below for men and 50 or below in women is considered too low, and a risk factor for heart disease.

While the numbers might be an indication that something in our bodies needs our attention, we shouldn't immediately jump to the conclusion that our heart is at risk.

Conditions such as pre-diabetes or untreated diabetes, pregnancy or lactation, liver conditions, low thyroid, and stress also have an impact on our cholesterol profile. Cholesterol numbers should be viewed as a small part of a big picture, not just as ominous warnings about heart disease.

Cholesterol is actually in our bodies to act as a defense in an inflammatory situation. (Remember—inflammation is caused by carbohydrates, not fat.) As inflammation causes lesions in a wall of an artery, the body responds by temporarily coating the lesions with cholesterol. If the inflammation improves, the cholesterol moves on so that the lesion can be repaired. Most of the time, however, the inflammatory condition continues unchecked (because we keep eating the bad stuff), and eventually the cholesterol is oxidized and ends up taking up more space in the artery, slowing arterial flow, and potentially breaking loose to form a clot. So the cholesterol didn't become an issue until the inflammatory condition had caused it to become oxidized.

Once again, the consequence of our modern way of eating is inflammation along with everything it brings, and the primal way to fight it is with liberal amounts of assorted fruits and vegetables, quality meat, fish and fish oils for the omega-3 fatty acids, and healthy fats.

Chapter 5

Getting Back To Basics

Although 500 generations may seem like an enormous expanse of time, in the grand scheme of things it's more like one page from an epic novel. After practicing the same way of life for over two million years, it was only 500 generations ago that our ancestors shifted the paradigm.

Suddenly (by historical standards), there came an end to the consumption of only wild and unprocessed food that they obtained through foraging and hunting in their own environment. Their search for food had been almost constant, impeded by harsh elements, and full of risk; moreover, success had never been guaranteed. Sometimes they had had days of feasting, but there were also times when they would suffer through periods of famine.

Culturally, we've come a long way from the days of our hunting-gathering-fishing ancestors as we have progressed through those 500 generations. In many ways, our lifestyles could be considered improved: we're safer, we're cleaner, we're more assured of finding food when we need it, we are even climate controlled.

Rather than venturing out into the wild, facing unknown hazards and stalking elusive prey, we venture into grocery stores, facing an array of delectable choices and stalking coupon specials or items on sale. While some hardy souls will partake of their meat in the raw state, more are likely to use their outdoor grills or even modernized spits to simulate the outdoor cooking habits of the caveman.

Our ancestors didn't have the choices we have in our time; they were limited by the availability of food sources in their own environment based on climate and geographic location; e.g., inland bands of our ancestors weren't consuming fish, and bands of people who lived in the colder regions didn't eat tropical vegetables and fruits. Now that we have so much more to choose from than our ancestors did, let's get back to choosing wisely.

If we try to imitate as much as possible the typical diet of Paleo man, researchers believe we stand a very good chance of obtaining the Paleo health and fitness. If we tweak our diets to consist mainly of meat, including organ meats such as liver and kidney, as well as fowl, fish, and shellfish, we'll have the building blocks for strength, vitality, and stamina.

We can still enjoy our eggs, too. They did—as many as they wanted—they'd never even heard of cholesterol. We also need to stop avoiding plant-derived foods and eat a good balance of fruit, vegetables, nuts (not peanuts—they're actually beans), and seeds. But if we really want Paleolithic health, we need to stop eating what they didn't eat: any kind of grains, beans, dairy products, potatoes, sugar, salt, processed food and the fat-loaded meats of domesticated animals. The post-Agricultural Revolution foods we've added are the basic cause of our dietary disaster.

Modern proponents of the Primal eating strategy assert that eating the foods for which we are genetically calibrated is the best way to keep our bodies at their healthiest and strongest. We get the optimum amount of protein, fat, amino acids, and some essential vitamins and minerals from our consumption of meat, and we get the necessary carbohydrates, fiber, and more vitamins and minerals from the plants we consume.

Our human genome, as it has developed over millions of years of evolution, determines our needs regarding nutrition and activity. Our bodies are adapted genetically and metabolically to process food from both animal and plant sources. For example, humans have a requirement for Vitamin B-12, but we can't reliably get it from eating only plant foods, so we must have some animal sources of food in our diet. In addition, our digestive systems produce specific enzymes to digest proteins found in animal tissue, shellfish, and insects (more than half the world's human population is estimated to eat a variety of insects). That's more than enough evidence that we were designed to be meat eaters.

Anecdotal evidence abounds of benefits gained from following this lifestyle. Faithful followers have shared detailed accounts of more effective weight loss, improved muscle tone, higher energy levels, increased immunity, and healthier skin. More impressive is reduced risk of diseases such as diabetes, heart disease, cancer, and arthritis. Even sufferers of MS have confirmed that their symptoms were alleviated when they followed the Paleo diet.

Chapter 6

Ancient Exercise And Rest Patterns

No good discussion of the Paleo lifestyle would be complete without addressing the exercise/rest patterns of our ancient ancestors. Obviously, it was not a sedentary lifestyle; however, it wasn't a grueling, constant grind, either. While Paleo man had to exert himself pretty hard to stay alive, this exertion was balanced with resting, socializing, playing, and low-level labor.

For Paleo man, there was no such thing as an exercise "routine." He would probably wake up every morning asking himself the question, "Need food?"

If the answer was no, he would have a low level exercise day; maybe he would work on the tools or weapons, dry some meat from the previous day's kill, gather firewood and other materials, or just sit around with the other men, swapping stories. (In the later Paleolithic years, he'd illustrate his stories by painting on his cave walls.) When the sun went down, he would get a full night's sleep so that he would be able to wake up the next morning and ask the question, "Need food?"

If the answer was yes, he needed to prepare himself for a hunt. The first thing he had to do was to find his quarry. This involved walking, sometimes for long distances, until he spotted his target. If it was small, like a rabbit or a squirrel, he might have to sneak up on it and club it or spear it, or perhaps he would have to sprint after it for some distance, hoping to corner it and get it that way.

Large, strong, fast animals presented a different challenge. If he wasn't able to catch them unaware and stun them with a blow so that they could be killed, they would run. This is where Paleo man really got his workout, and ironically, it's also where he had the advantage over the faster, stronger animal. Fortunately for him, humans had lost their body hair at this point; after all, we had evolved to the point where we had a larger brain, and could work out a way to keep ourselves warm in cold temperatures. Nature continued to help us out in warmer conditions by giving us the ability to cool ourselves off through the process of perspiration.

Animals, with their smaller brains, need a little more help from Nature, so they have fur coats to insulate them from the cold. Naturally, all that fur tends to be a little problematic when the weather warms up, especially if the animal decides to engage in any activity. Animals can't perspire, so their method of managing their temperature is by panting. The problem is, they can only pant when they're stationary. This turns out to be a serious handicap in the game of Run for Your Life.

Once the hunter has located his quarry, the game begins. Most of the large animals he hunted could obviously outrun him, but at some point, the anatomical physiology of each would come into play. The animal, in gaining some distance from its pursuer, would become overheated and need to rest for a while, panting to cool off. This enabled Paleo man, whose stamina for running distances was greater than the animal's, to catch up. The animal usually had some strength left, though, and the chase was on again. This might have gone through several stages before the animal was overcome by fatigue or heat stroke, and Paleo man had his chance to kill the animal. Now all he had to do was lift the animal and carry the dead weight (excuse the pun), or drag it back to home ground. Easy day.

Obviously, Paleo man would never have needed a gym or a defined schedule to stay fit—he had life and all its challenges to keep him in shape. The pattern of his workout would depend on the day. He might start with weight-bearing exercises as he lifted logs or moved large rocks for building purposes. Or the weight-bearing exercise could come after an intense aerobic activity, as he carried his prize for miles to his waiting companions. On the other hand, he might spend most of the day walking over variable terrain, climbing hills and trees, searching for elusive prey. On many occasions, he would be likely to sprint after small animals. Activities such as throwing a rock or his spear, digging, and chopping would ensure that he had a full body workout.

As most of the physical activity involved long distance walking, with the odd sprint or heavy lift thrown in for good measure, ligaments and joints would have remained extremely strong and flexible, and muscles would have been quite lean (as opposed to a huge muscle-bound man along the lines of someone like Arnold Schwarzenegger in his prime). Large muscles would not necessarily be very practical, reduce flexibility and range of motion, while the joints and ligaments would remain strong to adapt to walking great distances over variable terrain. Imagine what a setback a simple twisted ankle would be to a hunter chasing its prey, or even worse, trying to escape from a hungry predator!

It could be pretty extreme, but Paleo man enjoyed plenty of leisure time to give his body time to rest and refuel. If he lived day after day with a demanding schedule like this, he would be more prone to fatigue and injury, and his survival could be threatened. Paleo man and his comrades couldn't afford to take these kinds of risks, so it's believed they alternated strenuous days with low-activity days, as well as plenty of social fun and games to relieve stress from the regular life-or-death situations they found themselves in.

Sadly, many of today's fitness enthusiasts have lost touch with the important concept of making time to rest and regenerate. These people subscribe to a routine of punishing activity where the more intense the exercise, the better the results. While intense exercise does have a powerful effect in heightening a person's aerobic capacity, it also has the detrimental effect of increasing chances for injury and illness as the intense exercise places stress on muscles, tendons, ligament, bone, joints, and even the immune system! This leads researchers to the conclusion that the most intense exercise should be limited to no more than two sessions per week.

Regular physical activity does a lot of good for a body, but taking it to the extreme as we do in marathons, ultra-marathons, triathlons and other athlons—even extremely long distance bicycling competitions--are in opposition to the fitness regimen that our ancestors practiced. There's really no way to know how much distance the ancient hunter gatherers covered in a hunt, but studies among modern hunter gatherer cultures like the Aché tribe in Paraguay have revealed that the average distance covered by the most active hunters is only around 8-10km. Of course most of this would be walking distance – running for 10km to hunt an animal, only to come back empty-handed could leave the energy reserves so low that the result could almost be fatal with no other fuel readily available.

It's evident that our genetic adaptations have programmed us for a range of different activities, alternating between mild, moderate, and intense, for moderate amounts of time. Engaging in extremely high-intensity endurance exercise for more than a few hours has been shown to cause damage to joints, muscles, and the muscular tissue of the heart. In fact, studies have shown that the physiological and biochemical stress of such intense prolonged aerobic activity can actually increase the risk of cardio-vascular issues. Documented evidence has found signs of myocardial damage in runners immediately after finishing a marathon.

Other studies have found similar levels of coronary calcium in middle aged marathon runners and non-runners who had high risk factor of cardiovascular disease. Follow-up studies showed that their risk for a coronary event was similar to the coronary disease group. Further evaluative studies of top long-distance competitive runners revealed scarring in the heart muscle, and animal models have demonstrated an increased susceptibility to myocardial fibrosis and ventricular arrhythmias after endurance-type activity.

Note that the Paleo strategy does not recommend giving up exercise; not by any means. Our DNA legacy calls for a sensible regimen of exercise on a regular basis punctuated by periods of rest and leisure. Besides the benefits moderate exercise has on our muscular, skeletal, and cardiovascular system, it also impacts our insulin sensitivity as our muscles burn the stored glycogen during and after our workout. If we make it part of our lifestyle to move more during our day, we will stimulate effective metabolism of fat, strengthen our cardiovascular and immune systems, and fortify ourselves for the times when we step up to more intense workouts. We are designed for movement, not a sedentary life sitting in the office, the car, or on the couch!

Occasional sprinting doesn't usually cause the risk of burnout that excessive sustained aerobic exercise tends to produce, plus it helps to promote the production of Human Growth Hormone (HGH) and testosterone (in men), benefitting total fitness and delaying the deterioration of aging. Adding weight lifting sessions to the regimen stimulates development of lean muscle, hastens fat loss, and increases energy. Mixing the two types of workouts, aerobics and resistance training, is the best type of program to follow for building and toning muscle, losing fat, improving heart health, and maintaining overall good health.

The more spontaneous and intuitive we can keep our exercise schedule, the closer we'll be to following the basic lifestyle of our ancestors. Instead of saying things like, "Time to hit the gym," focus more on, "I feel like riding my bike to work today," or "This is a really nice day; I think I'll call (insert friend's name here) and go for a nice hike in the mountains." Avoiding anything that resembles a regimented schedule will make our fitness plan seem more natural, spontaneous, and pleasurable. We can still challenge ourselves with high intensity workouts; just keep them less frequent and more sensible. After all, the whole point is to add extra days to our lives, so why would we want to spend them in exhaustion?

Let's not forget the impact that exercise has on our stress levels. Paleo-man faced plenty of stress, but it was entirely different from the types of stress Modern man faces. While we might be anxious about deadlines, traffic, relationships, money, etc., Paleo man mostly had to deal with avoiding death. Sometimes it was a minute-to-minute kind of stress, where he was confronted with a hungry animal and had to instantly call upon every ounce of energy, speed, and strength to survive.

We've heard it before—the "fight or flight" response. His body automatically shut down any nonessential operations and released its emergency hormones, adrenaline and cortisol. His heart rate accelerated, pumping blood to his brain and putting it into high-alert mode so that he could respond immediately to the situation. The muscles in the rest of his body used the surge of energy-providing blood to physically react by running and jumping faster and higher than usual. Even his vision became more acute as his eyes dilated from the protective hormones. Once he survived this confrontation, no more stress. If he didn't survive—no more stress. In either case, he didn't have to suffer through days, weeks, and months of agonizing worry about the future.

Other types of stress that might last a little longer were situations where food or water was unavailable. This type of stress was easy to deal with as well. All he had to do was focus on filling the need. If he did, no more stress. If he didn't—well, at least he tried. Rest in peace. The point is, when Paleo man was confronted with stress, he had to deal with it at the moment and, one way or another, it was gone.

Nowadays, our stress doesn't seem to go away. When one problem is resolved, we find ourselves faced with two new ones. We still have the fight or flight hormones coming to aid us, but when we can't respond to resolve a problem immediately, stress chemicals build up in our bodies. We can't run because we're in our boss's office listening to him criticize our last project. We can't fight because—well, he's the boss and we need the job.

If we don't have the opportunity to burn off the stress, we can feel tired or even sick. Our body can react with high triglycerides, high LDL cholesterol and low HDL cholesterol, insulin resistance, and hypertension. If we accumulate any three of these conditions together, we have a condition called Metabolic Syndrome X. This can lead to an early heart attack.

This is about more than just losing weight or toning up—in this case, we have an actual bio-chemical need for exercise. We've got to deal with our stress chemicals on a daily basis by staying active.

If Paleo man did have any residual stress after his day's hunt, he had a built-in support group in his own Paleo network. Since he lived with family members and other adults he could trust, each homecoming was a virtual celebration—he had survived to see another day. It's hard to know for sure the types of activities they indulged in during their leisure time, but human nature tells us that they most likely spent time relaxing and, possibly playing.

If the hunt had been successful, they would feast—sometimes for days. Modern hunter gatherer tribes have formal celebrations that include music and dancing. These are forms of self-expression, and humans have a need for self-expression, so it's not too far-fetched to believe that our ancestors might have had some music and movement in their lives. Some of the more creative members of the tribe probably even invented some games where everyone could participate.

This type of community life was undoubtedly very beneficial to everyone, but it was an ideal way for children to grow up. It's difficult to know whether all children recognized one set of parents as their own, or believed that every adult in the community played a parenting role. In either case, there were plenty of adults available for the children to learn from. If a parent was lost for some reason, there were still other "parents" who could undertake the role of guardian—individuals trusted by everyone in the community. Food, exercise, leisure, and security—that was the Paleo way of life.

Chapter 7

Connecting the Past to Our Future

In wrapping up any discussion of the Paleo or Primal lifestyle, we shouldn't overlook the criticisms from those who would challenge the concept; specifically the previously mentioned idea that the premise of the diet is unfounded. Detractors will insist that we can't claim the people in the Paleolithic period were free of the diseases we've mentioned because they didn't live long enough to develop any of them.

While it may be true that archaeologists haven't made many discoveries of fossilized remains that indicate a long life-span, it's also true that they've only uncovered a mere fraction of artifacts to represent the population. We know that many people from this era died at a young age, in fact the average life span at the time was 33*. Discoveries continue to be made, and there has been remains found of a Paleolithic man that lived to the age of 94, so it may not be as rare as we might think.

In the meantime, we actually have living hunter gatherer societies to study. People in isolated cultures like the natives of the Tokelau Islands can show us how a Paleo-style diet affects human health. Away from the influence of civilization, the typical diet of Tokelau inhabitants consisted primarily of coconut, with over 50% of what they ate being (mostly saturated) fat. The only health problems the people suffered were skin diseases, asthma, and infectious diseases like measles, chicken pox, and leprosy.

In the 1970s, civilization infringed on the Islands, bringing trading posts, a cash economy, and foods from the outside. As a result, the consumption of coconut diminished, and sugar consumption increased by 32kg per year per person. Canned meats, frozen foods, and bread products became part of their diet, and they increased their alcohol and tobacco consumption.

It wasn't long before the Islanders began to experience diabetes, heart disease, gout, high blood pressure, and cancer. They started to gain weight, an increase of 10-15kgs in both men and women. In people who had volunteered to move from the islands to civilized communities in New Zealand, the changes in health were even more dramatic, with exceptionally high frequency of the same diseases.

That's pretty solid evidence that our modern diet has a devastating impact on our health. If the islanders had remained innocent of the ways and the diet of the modern world, they most likely would have escaped this physical deterioration. The intrusion of the modern world on the people of the Tokelau Islands had the same effect on them as the Agricultural Revolution had on our ancient ancestors.

* * * * *

The agricultural revolution introduced grains, legumes, dairy products, and sugar to our species, and now the Paleo diet eliminates them. Our focus should be on unprocessed, natural foods. Obviously, evolution and modern technology have combined to alter the food supply, so it's not possible to precisely replicate the Paleo way of eating. Technology has improved dramatically and with lightning speed throughout the past 10,000 years, however evolution is a much longer and slower process, and our bodies are fighting a losing battle to keep up with the changes. But if we make an effort to ensure that our protein is obtained from natural sources such as wild-caught fish, free range chicken and eggs, and grass-fed meat, we're at least approximating the caveman protein consumption.

The rest of our diet should feature seasonal vegetables and fruits (locally grown, when possible), as well as healthy fats from avocados, nuts, olive oils, and coconut oil. As much as we're able, we should avoid dairy products, processed foods, trans-fats, grains, legumes, starchy vegetables like potatoes, added salt, and sugar.

The important thing to remember is that the Paleo diet is just a part of a lifestyle; a diet alone is not necessarily enough to ensure that modern humans can acquire the superior level of health that our ancestors enjoyed. By combining the diet with other considerations such as a regular, sensible exercise program, stress management, sufficient amounts of sleep, reasonable exposure to the sun, avoidance of tobacco smoke, and reduced contact with pollutants, we should all take the health and happiness of the past well into our future, for the benefit of our own quality of life, as well as our kids and future generations.

* *Life expectancy* – According to Wikipedia, life expectancy during the Paleolithic era (2.5 million years ago to 10,000 B.C.) was around 33, which factored in the high rates of infant death. If children made it to puberty then life expectancy increase up to the age of 39 and if they managed to reach 39 they could expect to live until 54. This is a fit, strong and lean 54, not someone struggling to hang on for dear life. Major causes of death in those days were entirely primitive: predators, accidents or infections… not heart disease, diabetes or obesity.

While an average age of 33 sounds quite low to us, the advent of agriculture and civilization caused life expectancy to drop significantly, reaching a low of 18 during the Bronze Age of 3,300 B.C. – 1,200 B.C. Life expectancy remained between 20 and 30 right through to about 1,500 A.D., and then climbed only gradually, reaching about 30 in 1800, and about 40-50 in 1900 in the more developed countries. The past century has seen a dramatic increase in life expectancy mainly due to advances in medicine, allowing us to limit infant mortality rates and prevent disease plagues.

Chapter 8

Becoming The Caveman (Or Woman) Of The Future

This Paleo/Primal Diet premise is based on millions of years of human evolution and scientific evidence. Men before me have paved the way for sharing this knowledge, and credit must go to Dr Loren Cordain, Robb Wolf, and Mark Sisson, among others, who have gone out and researched and published much of the information provided here. Much of their research is based on our genetics, and the use of skeletal evidence for their findings. Fad diets come and go, but how can you argue with millions of years of human evolution?

I cannot claim to have a PhD in nutrition, my background is as a chef, and more recently a personal trainer, and as someone who is dedicated to helping people rid themselves of obesity, as well as the many diseases and problems that come with it.

A great deal of research and practical application has gone into the making of this book, and resources are provided at the end for your convenience. I urge you to carry a healthy amount of skepticism and go out and follow up with your own research as well. Most importantly, I urge you to take action, and in the final chapter I will provide some of my favourite recipes that can be made on a day-to-day basis at home, as well as some very simple action steps for improving your foundation of fitness, no matter what your current starting point now is.

I know that the first couple of weeks of trying something new like this can be challenging, as you work out what you should and shouldn't eat, where to look for food, how to prepare for times when you are going out to dinner, or away from home where you have much less control over what you can eat. Here are a couple of suggestions to put it all in perspective, and hopefully make the transition to a healthier Paleo lifestyle a lot easier for you.

Remember that it takes 21 days of doing the same thing over and over before it becomes a habit. That's 3 weeks that you would need to be consistently "hunting and gathering" your new food sources. If you feel happy that this Paleo diet just makes sense, and you're prepared to jump straight into the deep end and giving it a try, that's fantastic. If however, this all seems a bit overwhelming and you want to try it in smaller chunks, how about this for a simple suggestion…

Week 1 – Replace one meal, for example breakfast, each day for the week, whilst eating normally for the rest of the day.

Week 2 – Keep eating a Paleo style breakfast each day, and add one more meal, like lunch.

Week 3 – By this point, you could already be starting to notice some changes in the way you feel. Not necessarily any dramatic weight changes just yet, but all in good time! This week is when you should feel quite comfortable creating every meal of the day as a Paleo meal.

Poor food choices tend to lead to a downward spiral, and it can be a vicious cycle to break out of. The opposite is also true, by having at least one healthy meal each day, it will lead to a more positive cycle. Get a vitamin-rich breakfast, and you should get a good boost of energy to start the day, which could lead to you getting the urge to go for a long walk, or a short jog, which could then lead you to want a healthy snack that doesn't weigh you down and make you feel bloated, so that you have more energy to do it again, and so on it could continue. The key here is some persistence, and tuning in to how your body feels and responds to the fuel you feed it.

Super Tip – If there is ever anything in your diet that you're unsure about whether it is good for you or not, here is the simplest way to find out. Remove the item (eg; grains, dairy, alcohol) from your diet for 2 weeks, and then re-introduce it. If it doesn't make you feel any different, then it is good for you. If you re-introduce a food and it has some sort of effect on your body, then it's probably not good for you to eat, or at the very least is making your body work a lot harder to break it down. You can apply this to absolutely anything, try it for yourself!

I titled this chapter *"Becoming The Caveman (Or Cavewoman) Of The Future"*, not because I expect you to go out and live in a cave, fashion a spear for hunting and learn how to make fire by rubbing two sticks together, but because I think you are capable enough and strong enough to make the best of both worlds.

Fast foods and convenience foods are everywhere, you don't have to look very hard, and modern technology has given us great comfort and security, but the cost has been high. We have become soft, lazy, and more reliant on gadgets and other people to think and do the work for us.

It's not all bad though, as food is far more abundant and readily available for us at the local shop, it's simply a matter of making a better choice. Bypass the bakery, the McDonalds, and even the supermarkets, and head for the local butcher, and the organic fruit and veg shops instead. Even better still, hunt out your local farmer, or find a farmers market in your local area that provide organic vegetables, wild-caught seafood and grass-fed meats.

We can even use much of our modern technology to improve our fitness, instead of spending all day sitting at the computer desk, sitting in the car or on the train, and sitting on the couch at home, and in the next chapter I'll give you some simple suggestions on how…

Chapter 9

Exercise For The Paleo Lifestyle

When it comes to achieving your ideal body weight goals, I believe that about 20% of it is exercise, while the other 80% is what you actually eat. Yes, it's that important! Before I get onto the recipes (which by the way, should help you take the first action step and also to realize that diets are not all about restricting yourself to tasteless horrible foods!), I just want to show you how to increase your base level of fitness to lose weight, gain strength, and feel great!

You've probably seen the ads by local government about "Find 30" etc, which is their basic recommendation to find 30 minutes per day to exercise. While this is a nice thought, I honestly don't think they go far enough with their minimum recommendations. Before you start freaking out about forking out tons of money for a gym membership and spending every spare waking minute pumping out kilometers on the treadmills or bikes, allow me to explain.

When you think of exercise, it generally conjures up thoughts of heavy panting, red faces, and dripping with sweat, from jogging, or cycling, or whatever other activity they may be doing, in an attempt to reach that "runners high". As we know from studying our history, this is not really the best way for us to exercise, as Paleo man would have rarely if ever run or jogged 10 or 20km.

Walking is the best way to go, especially if you're at a less than ideal starting point. Paleo man, like many other animals in nature, would have conserved energy by stalking his prey until he got close enough, and then a quick sprint to attack may be all that was needed to take down the prey with his weapons. Think about any other carnivore in nature (and yes, we are still part of the Animal Kingdom, although humans are technically omnivores) such as cheetahs, lions, tigers, snakes etc.

Let's take a quick look at our own bodies, and what walking can do for us. It is often not intense enough to bring our large leg muscles into use, however the great thing is that our ligaments still get worked. Quite a lot actually. Even professional athletes often break down at the joints because they can focus too much on building up muscle strength and not enough on strong ligaments.

Here's why – when we perform any action, our brain sends signals to that part of the body, and recruits the muscles or ligaments that it thinks it will need to perform the function required. It will always go for whatever is the least necessary to perform the function in order to conserve energy. In other words, if it only needs to pick up a light weight of 1kg it may only recruit the tendons in the wrist, whereas if you were to pick up a 60kg dumbbell, you will require significantly more muscles in order to lift the weight.

With that in mind, walking long distances each day is an excellent way to improve your joint strength, even though you may not necessarily feel like it's been a proper workout. You may be surprised to know however, that you can also increase your cardio fitness just through walking. This is where I disagree with the government recommendations, and you should aim for 1-2 hours of walking each day.

Of course, this may be quite challenging to begin with, but even if you started with 30 minutes per day and built up to 1 or 2 hours, it would be a great place to start. Definitely don't limit yourself to any government recommendations, these are usually absolute minimum amounts to go for.

This is also a fantastic way for you to get started, even if you have joint problems like arthritis, or dealing with weight issues that make jogging impossible because of the added strain put on the joints. Even better, walk on slightly uneven surfaces like gravel or cobblestones, and see how quickly you can improve your ankle stability too! In a practical sense, you can use modern technology to aid you as I mentioned earlier… a treadmill at home in front of the tv, breaking up the daily commute by getting off a couple of stops early and walking, and you can even get a treadmill put in at work so you can walk and work on the computer at the same time!

Keeping in mind that walking long distances is an excellent starting point, once you feel comfortable it's time to add in an occasional sprint, and some heavy lifting. Sprinting is all about short, sharp bursts of energy. Mark out a distance, chase a ball, or find some other target to race at, and go for it! Sprinting might sound like hard work, but if you give yourself a challenge to aim for, and plenty of rest in between, it can be lot's of fun, and can also be a really quick way to bring on that "runners high"! Any sort of ball sport can be good for this, even just throwing a frisbee around with a friend.

Finally, when it comes to lifting heavy objects, think about the sort of things that Paleo man may have done, like thrown a spear, picked up rocks or large branches for shelter, climbed up trees, or carrying a large dead animal back to camp.

Mix up your exercise for variety, don't stick to the same routine. Not only will this help prevent boredom, but also burnout. Your body needs new challenges thrown at it all the time. If you do the same workout 3 times per week, your body will just get used to it, and your fitness will plateau.

What can be even more important than the exercise you do, is what you don't do, or in other words, how much rest you get. Paleo man had huge challenges to overcome on some days, and the stress of an attack by a predator would be enough to send the heart rate sky-high. But at the times when food was plentiful and shelter had been built, there would have been much time to socialize with family and friends, and probably even play games, and come up with other forms of entertainment such as art.

These rest periods are crucial to recover and regenerate muscles to full capacity. Too many people these days exercise until they can't move, and then suffer from soreness for days afterwards. If Paleo man woke up feeling stiff, sore, and hungry, his chances of a successful hunt would be greatly reduced. Here's a useful guideline to follow – if you're tired and don't feel like exercising, then don't. If you feel full of energy and ready to attack the day, then get out there and have some fun!

Chapter 10

Paleo Recipes For Good Health

This is the section that will help you take what you've just learnt, and put it into action straight away with some healthy eating ideas. Not only that, I want to show you that eating healthy does not necessarily mean that you have to lose out on taste, or even quantity. By removing things like grains from your diet, you're removing the "filler" items of meals, things like bread which help to fill you up, but don't provide any decent nutrition.

If you were to have a sandwich, for example, and removed the bread, all you'll be left with is the meat and salad on the inside. Add a little bit of healthy fat, fill up on that, and your body will naturally tell you when it's time to stop eating, and without the sugar spike (and crash) that comes from eating the carbs!

Anyway, it's time to get right into the good stuff…

Egg Muffins

I tend to do a lot of cooking on a Sunday to prepare for the rest of the week, and these brilliant muffins can be made in advance to heat up for a quick and easy breakfast later in the week. Very versatile, you can add pretty much any ingredients you like, and to save on cleaning up after you could even make a frittata by mixing it all together in a cake dish rather than muffin trays!

A little coconut milk (about ½ cup) can be optionally added if you need more liquid, which may seem strange at first, but as long as you don't put too much in it won't overpower the tastebuds with that coconut flavour, and you might find it actually does work quite well.

Ingredients:

Butter, Coconut oil, or Olive oil (for greasing the tin)

12 eggs

1 onion, finely diced

1 red capsicum, finely diced

500g minced meat, cooked (beef, pork, kangaroo, whatever takes your fancy)

Sea salt and pepper, for seasoning

MAKES APPROXIMATELY 12 MUFFINS (OR 1 LARGE FRITTATA TRAY)

How To Make Egg Muffins:

Preheat oven to 180C (360F).

Grease 12 muffin tins with butter or oil, or you can even line with baking paper cups (which also help them to keep their shape).

In a bowl, beat the eggs. Add the optional ½ cup of coconut milk if you wish.

Add the cooked meat, along with the onion, capsicum and seasoning. Carefully ladle or spoon into muffin tins.

Bake for approximately 18-20 minutes in the oven. You can tell when it's cooked by sticking a knife into the muffin, if it comes out clean it's ready!

Zucchini Bake

This is pretty simple to make, is full of goodness and flavour, and can be eaten hot or cold. Serve for dinner with a salad, and you can even make it in advance to heat up later.

Ingredients:

4 tablespoons of butter

1 medium onion, finely diced

1kg zucchini, grated

300g minced meat (beef, pork, lamb, or any other that you have available)

3 eggs, beaten

Sea salt and pepper, for seasoning

SERVES 4

How To Make Zucchini Bake:

Preheat oven to 180C (360F).

In a pan over medium heat, melt the butter and add onion and zucchini. Saute lightly until zucchini is tender, about 5-7 minutes should do it. Put zucchini in a colander to drain off any excess liquid.

Add the minced meat to the pan, and sauté until browned. Combine the meat and zucchini in a bowl and season to taste. Add eggs, mix well, and pour into a casserole dish or deep pan.

Bake uncovered for about 35-40 minutes, or until slightly browned and you can stick a knife in and pull it out clean.

Aussie Beef Burger

While the burger tends to be a very common food item in the US, here in Australia we've long had our own twist on this simple meal by serving it with fried egg to pack an extra hit of protein, and beetroot. While you can add pretty much anything you like to a burger, the big difference with this recipe here is that we won't be having it in a bun, as bread is a no-no.

However, you can roast a big field mushroom and serve it open, or even wrap it up in some cos or iceberg lettuce just for something a bit different.

Ingredients:

500g minced beef (or pork, or lamb, or even kangaroo)

1 clove of garlic, crushed

2 tablespoons of fresh lemon juice

1 teaspoon of finely chopped oregano

2 tablespoons finely chopped flat-leaf parsley

¼ teaspoon ground cumin

¼ teaspoon ground pepper

1 medium plum tomato, crushed

1 small red onion, sliced

4 slices of beetroot

4 fried eggs

Optional extras – roasted field mushroom (without stalk), avocado and lettuce

SERVES 4

How To Make Aussie Beef Burgers

Mix together the minced meat, lemon juice, oregano, cumin, tomato and parsley. Make 4 burger patties, about 2cm thick.

Grill burgers for about 5 minutes on each side, or until cooked, on a hot pan or hotplate. (If you're having field mushrooms, cook them in the oven for about 5-7 minutes at 180C, and fry the eggs, while the burgers are cooking on the grill).

Place either field mushroom or burger at the base, then top with beetroot, egg, onion, and any other toppings you might like to add.

NOTE: The egg is best fried with the yolk still slightly runny, so that the juices ooze out over the burger as you eat.

Chorizo Con Huevos

There are many ways to cook eggs, and they make a fantastic way to start the day for breakfast. Many of them don't really require a recipe, just a little bit of creativity in how you want to use them. Scrambled eggs with slices of avocado and smoked salmon is an excellent way to get protein, good fats, and omega-3, while this particular recipe will spice things up a bit with some Spanish-style chorizo sausage!

Ingredients:

8 eggs, beaten

1 tablespoon olive oil

500g Chorizo sausage

1 medium onion, diced

2 chillies, finely chopped

1 tablespoon coriander, finely chopped

1 large avocado, mashed

SERVES 4

How To Make Chorizo Con Huevos

Heat the oil in a frying pan over medium heat, then add the chorizo. Use a fork or spatula to break up the meat as it cooks, be careful not to allow oil to spit up at you.

Brown the chorizo, then drain any excess oil. Add the onions and cook till translucent (see-through).

Add the chillies and cook for an extra minute or two, before adding the egg mixture. Stir the eggs while cooking to give it a scrambled effect.

Add the coriander just at the end of cooking, and serve with avocado, and goes great with a salsa if you happen to have one handy.

Granny Apple Muffins

One of the trickiest things you may find with eating Paleo is a good snack to eat, particularly when you travel lots or if you're really short of time. These muffins are a great snack, I enjoy having them with breakfast as well, you can make them in advance, and are great warm or cold!

If you don't like mucking around with muffin tins, you can even cook them in a tray and make them as a slice. It's not easy to come across Paleo-friendly muffins or cakes, but these little beauties are a winner every time.

Ingredients:

Butter, for greasing the tin

2 ½ cups almond flour

1 large apple, peeled, cored and grated (Granny Smith apples are best)

2 cups carrots, peeled and grated

1 tablespoon cinnamon

2 teaspoons baking soda

1 cup coconut, shredded

1 cup of raisins

3 large eggs

½ teaspoon sea salt

2 tablespoons of honey (optional)

½ cup coconut or avocado oil

1 teaspoon vanilla extract

MAKES ABOUT 10-12 MUFFINS

How To Make Granny Apple Muffins

Preheat oven to 180C (360F), and grease your muffin tins well with butter.

In a large bowl, combine almond flour, cinnamon, baking soda, carrot, apple, coconut, raisins and salt.

In a separate bowl, whisk together the eggs, honey, oil and vanilla extract. Pour this mixture over the dry ingredients and mix well. This should make quite a thick batter.

Spoon the batter into the muffin tins and cook in the oven for 40-50 minutes. It's ready when you can insert a skewer or knife into the muffin and remove it clean.

Leave muffins to cool for 8-10 minutes, then transfer to a cake rack to finish cooling.

Kangaroo Kofta Balls

Kangaroo is certainly a favourite meat to be eaten in Australia, it's very lean, is high in protein and full of flavour. If you're upset that eating Paleo will mean you might have to miss out on your favourite spaghetti and meatballs, then I'm sure that this dish will more than make up for it!

If you do happen to have any leftovers (it's unlikely, but you never know), then this can be enjoyed with a breakfast scramble the next day, or is even great cold as a handy snack. You can also make this with any other kind of meat, such as beef, pork, lamb, bison, goat, or whatever else may be available locally.

Ingredients:

1 tablespoon butter

½ cup spring onions, finely chopped

1 cup mushrooms, finely chopped

1kg minced kangaroo meat

¼ cup fresh parsley, finely chopped

1 egg, beaten

2 tablespoons lemon zest

½ tablespoon oregano

¼ cup olive oil

¼ cup crushed tomatoes

2 tablespoons red wine

1 garlic clove, crushed

¼ teaspoon ground cinnamon

Sea salt and pepper, for seasoning

SERVES 4

How To Make Kangaroo Kofta Balls

Melt butter in a frying pan over medium heat. Add the spring onions and sauté until tender.

Transfer to a large bowl and add mushrooms, kangaroo, parsley, egg and lemon zest to bowl with spring onions.

Season with sea salt, pepper and oregano, and mix all the ingredients together well. Allow to stand in refrigerator for 1 hour.

Form balls with the meat mixture, roughly about the size of a golf ball and set aside.

Add olive oil to the same frying pan, and heat over a medium-high heat.

Cook meatballs in batches if your pan is not big enough to carry them all. Brown evenly on all sides, and then place on paper towel to drain any excess oil. Once they are all cooked, transfer them to a serving dish.

Add the wine, crushed tomatoes, garlic and cinnamon to the frying pan. Cook until well blended, and season with sea salt and pepper if necessary.

Pour the sauce over the meatballs, and serve with toothpicks.

Cauliflower Mush

I was going to call this cauliflower mash, but it turns out to be really more of a mush in the end. Don't let that fool you though, as it still tastes fantastic. Normally I wouldn't put cauliflower and tasty in the same sentence together, but in this case it's an excellent way to eat a vitamin-rich vegetable, and it can go with just about anything!

It's also another excellent recipe that can be made in advance and kept aside for future meals.

Ingredients:

I head of fresh cauliflower, grated (or use a food processor)

4 cups (1L) of chicken stock

1 cup almond meal

Sea salt and pepper, for seasoning

How To Make Cauliflower Mush

In a large saucepan, mix together the grated cauliflower, almond meal and chicken over a medium heat.

Bring to the boil, then cover and reduce the heat to simmer for about 20 minutes, stirring occasionally until all the liquid is absorbed.

Season with sea salt and pepper, and serve on the side of any meal you like. Enjoy!

Schweet Potato Roschtis

If you're having a hard time accepting that eating potato is no longer an option (if you're being strict on yourself that is), then this makes for an excellent alternative. Full of nutrition and energy, and another recipe that can pretty much go on the side of any other dish you're making, these are also really quick and easy to make.

You can get fancy and make these really small and serve as canapés at a cocktail party, or go crazy and shape big hamburger sized ones, the choice is yours. I love a good bit of spice, but you can omit the cumin and cayenne pepper if it's a bit too much for you to handle.

Ingredients:

2 tablespoons olive oil (or coconut, or avocado oil)

500g sweet potato, peeled and grated

3 teaspoons cumin

1 teaspoon cayenne pepper

2 eggs, beaten

1 cup almond meal

Sea salt and pepper, for seasoning

How To Make Schweet Potato Roschtis

In a large bowl, mix the beaten egg, almond meal, cumin, cayenne pepper, salt and pepper into the grated sweet potato.

Form patties flattened out in your hands. Around half the size of your palm is a good amount to work with.

Heat the oil in a frying pan over a medium-high heat, and fry the patties for about 3-5 minutes on each side. Depending on size, it may be a good idea to finish them off in a hot oven for a couple of minutes, and serve hot.

Chicken Cacciatore

This is one of my favourite chicken dishes to make, as it's so tasty and full of protein with the goodness of vegetables. Cacciatore is basically a chicken stew, and can be made in a variety of ways. I like to use chicken thighs as they are very tender and will absorb more of the surrounding flavours of the dish, but any part of the chicken can be used. Feel free to add any other seasonal vegetables available to give yourself a bit of variety.

It can all be made in one pot, so cleaning up afterwards is a lot easier, and you can make a larger batch in advance to heat up when needed, which is great if you know you have a busy week ahead!

Ingredients:

2 tablespoons Extra-Virgin Olive oil

8 (approx. 1.5kg) chicken thigh cutlets

1 red onion, sliced

200g button mushrooms, sliced

1 red capsicum, sliced

4 slices pancetta, roughly chopped

2 garlic cloves, crushed

1 cup Kalamata (black) olives, pitted and sliced

400ml (1 can) crushed tomatoes

½ cup red wine

¼ cup oregano leaves, roughly chopped

¼ cup fresh basil, roughly chopped

Sea salt and pepper, for seasoning

SERVES 4

How To Make Chicken Cacciatore

In a large saucepan, heat the oil over a medium-high heat. Add the chicken and brown the outsides.

Remove chicken from the heat, and add the onion and pancetta. Cook until the onion becomes translucent.

Return the chicken back to the pot, along with the garlic, mushrooms and capsicum. Cook for a further 2-3 minutes, or until the mushroom and capsicum softens.

Add the olives and the red wine, and cook till the red wine reduces by half. This will increase the richness and intensity of the flavour.

Add the crushed tomatoes, and allow it to simmer on a low heat for at least 15-20 minutes. If the sauce becomes too thick you can add a little water to improve the consistency.

Finally, in the last minute or two of cooking, add the basil, oregano, and season with sea salt and pepper.

Hot And Spicy Fried Chicken

Forget the Colonel, you can make your own fried chicken at home… and you can even say that it's good for you! By using a quality fresh oil like coconut oil for cooking, you can avoid the horrendous trans-fats that fast food places (I can't bring myself to call them "restaurants") regularly use.

The Colonel has his secret recipe of herbs and spices, but you can mix and match anything you have on the spice rack at home to make a different and delicious flavour combination that your kids will surely be drooling over.

You'll need a pair of tongs, slotted spoon or spatula for moving and turning the chicken, and try to keep the handling down to a minimum or you may find the outer coating with all the flavour-some goodness falls off into the pan!

Ingredients:

1 cup (250ml) coconut oil

1kg chicken pieces

2 large eggs, beaten

1 cup almond flour

1 teaspoon paprika

1 teaspoon cayenne pepper

1 teaspoon Cajun spice

½ teaspoon sea salt

½ teaspoon cracked black pepper

½ teaspoon dried thyme

½ teaspoon dried basil

SERVES 4

How To Make Hot And Spicy Fried Chicken

Heat the coconut oil in a large frying pan over high heat. Preheat oven to 200C (400F).

Combine all the dry ingredients (almond flour, herbs and spices) in a large bowl and mix well.

Place the chicken in the beaten egg mixture, then coat well in the dry mixture. Place in the hot oil, and cook till both sides are browned (about 2 minutes each side).

Place a drying rack on your oven tray, and spread the chicken out across the rack so each piece of chicken has some space in between.

Put the tray of chicken in the oven to cook for a further 10-15 minutes. Use a skewer to pierce the skin of a chicken, if the fluid runs clear it's ready to go, if it still looks pink or red, it needs a bit longer in the oven.

NOTE: If you have trouble keeping the dry mixture sticking to the chicken, roll the pieces in a little flour before dipping into the beaten egg, as this should help it stick. Line your oven baking tray with aluminium foil to make it a bit easier to clean later.

Barramundi Semi-Poached In White Wine Sauce

Barramundi is a magnificent fish caught around the top-end of Australia, and it has a very soft, buttery type of flesh. This recipe will work well with just about any sort of fish, with a creamy white wine sauce that adds an extra dimension of flavour.

Of course, always try to find wild-caught fish for the extra load of omega-3, even if it is a bit more expensive it's worth it for the benefits to your health.

Ingredients:

2 x 200g fresh wild caught Barramundi fillet

1 tablespoon olive oil

20g unsalted butter

1 cup white wine

1 teaspoon fresh basil, roughly chopped

1 teaspoon fresh thyme, roughly chopped

Juice of 1 lemon

Sea salt and pepper, for seasoning

SERVES 2

How To Make Barramundi Semi-Poached In White Wine Sauce

Preheat oven to 180C (360F).

Heat olive oil in a medium oven-proof frying pan over a medium-high heat.

Add barramundi fillets to the hot frying pan (frying pan must be hot, or you will not get the nice caramelisation effect on the outside of the fish), and cook for about 3 minutes on each side.

Add the butter, white wine, lemon juice, basil, thyme and seasoning to the pan, and place in the oven to finish cooking. About 5 or 6 minutes in the oven should be enough, the flesh of the fish will flake away in large chunks when it is cooked and ready to eat.

Serve with some brightly coloured vegetables, a wedge of lemon, and a sprinkle of fresh parsley, and this will make a meal fit for a caveman! (Or even a romantic dinner).

Osso Buco

This is another very versatile stew type of meal, and is great for using up secondary cuts of meat if you need a cheaper option for dinner. You can easily replace the veal with lamb or beef shanks if you prefer. The longer you braise the meat for, the better it will taste, particularly to bring out the richness of the marrow hiding within the bone!

Ingredients:

4 thick veal shanks

¼ cup (60ml) coconut oil

2 brown onions, roughly chopped

1 large carrot, peeled and chopped

1 green capsicum, chopped

1 red capsicum, chopped

1 stick of celery, chopped

3 cloves of garlic, crushed

½ cup (125ml) of dry white wine

1 cup (250ml) chicken stock

Juice of 1 lemon

800ml (2 cans) crushed tomatoes

1 tablespoon fresh basil, roughly chopped

1 bay leaf

¼ teaspoon sea salt

1 teaspoon freshly cracked black pepper

2 sprigs of fresh thyme

SERVES 4

How To Make Osso Buco

Take meat out of refrigeration and allow it to come down to room temperature (for about 30 minutes). Season shanks well with a pinch of sea salt and black pepper.

Heat coconut oil over high heat in a large frying pan. Brown both sides of shanks for about 3 minutes on each side. Remove the meat and set aside.

Reduce the heat of the pan to medium-high, and preheat the oven to 170C (350F).

Saute the onions, carrots, capsicum, celery and garlic in the frying pan until they are slightly softened, about 5 minutes.

Increase the temperature to high and add the wine and chicken stock. Deglaze the pan as you add the lemon juice, tomatoes, basil, bay leaf, salt and pepper.

Reduce the liquid by about a third by cooking in the uncovered pan. At this point you can now return the shanks to the pot, and add the sprigs of thyme.

Cover with a lid or aluminium foil and place in the oven to braise for 1 ½ to 2 hours. Remove from the oven when the meat is cooked to very tender and almost falling off the bone.

Use a slotted spoon to carefully remove the meat and vegetables onto a serving plate. Continue cooking the sauce until you reduce it down to the desired thickness, and pour over the shanks to serve.

NOTE: You can also add a tablespoon of tomato paste if you want to increase the thickness and richness of the sauce.

Rich Chocolate Truffles

Dessert is an indulgence that many people give up when they go onto a diet, but it's not necessary. Not when you have options like dark chocolate, strawberries, blueberries and coconut milk to work with. For the best anti-oxidant results, use chocolate that is at least 70% cacao content.

These little beauties are pretty simple to make, but can get a bit time consuming and messy when shaping them into balls. I like to use two spoons and shape them more into an oval with three sides, by a method called Quenelle. This will help keep the messy hands to a minimum, particularly if you have a helper who likes to 'test' the recipe (ie; licking their fingers clean of chocolate when they should be making truffles!). These truffles tend to taste better the day after you make them, so don't be afraid to make them well in advance.

Ingredients:

400ml (1 can) full fat coconut milk

2 tablespoons coconut oil

500g Dark chocolate (minimum 70%), broken into small pieces

½ teaspoon vanilla extract

Cocoa powder

How To Make Rich Chocolate Truffles

Add the coconut milk and coconut oil to a saucepan on a medium-low heat, stirring until the coconut oil melts and the mixture comes to a light boil. Don't allow to come to a rolling boil, or you will have burnt milk. Remove from the heat.

Add the chocolate pieces to the coconut milk mixture and stir until all the chocolate is completely melted. Add the vanilla extract, and continue stirring until the chocolate thickens and cools down slightly.

Transfer mixture to a shallow dish and leave out to cool. After about an hour transfer the dish to the refrigerator to cool right down, and allow to thicken for at least 2 hours (overnight is fine).

Place some sifted cocoa powder into a shallow bowl or container. Remove the chocolate mixture from the fridge and allow to sit at room temperature for 5-10 minutes, until it reaches a clay-like consistency which is easier to work with.

Quenelle the chocolate by scooping up a small amount with a teaspoon, then use another teaspoon to scoop it around and knock the top off. Try and keep each one about the same size, but don't worry too much if they're not all perfectly rounded clones. Rolling them between the palms of your hands is fine too, but as previously mentioned, is a lot messier.

Finish them off by rolling them in the cocoa powder so they are lightly dusted. Refrigerate until needed.

NOTE: These keep well for quite a while, and can even be frozen. Substitute vanilla extract with any other flavouring of your choice, including liqueurs like Grand Marnier, and they also go great eaten with a fresh mint leaf. Optionally you can also replace the cocoa powder with finely chopped nuts if you like.

Pears Poached In Red Wine

Fruit makes for an excellent dessert if you still feel the need for something sweet after dinner (like I do!). Red wine is high in anti-oxidants, and by infusing it into pears as they poach, along with other spices full of macro-nutrients, this makes for quite a healthy treat.

These look spectacular, and the smell alone will fill your house with a delicious aroma as the pears simmer away in the background, which your guests will love, and help you to remember that you have them cooking on the stove! The main trick is to cook them until they are tender all the way through, and you can test with a skewer through the middle of the fruit.

Ingredients:

4 Pears, peeled and cored (leave the stem in the top though)

500ml dry red wine

1 tablespoon honey

2 whole star anise

2 cinnamon sticks

1 vanilla bean, split

SERVES 4

How To Make Pears Poached In Red Wine

Combine the wine, honey, star anise, cinnamon and vanilla bean in a saucepan over a medium heat, and cook, stirring, for about 2 minutes, or until the honey dissolves into the liquid.

Add the pears and bring to the boil. Reduce heat to low, and simmer pears for about 1 hour, or until they are tender enough. Turn the pears occasionally as they cook.

Remove from the heat and set aside for 10 minutes to cool.

Increase the heat of the saucepan and bring the syrup to a boil. Continue cooking for 10 minutes until the sauce thickens slightly. Pour syrup over the pears and set aside to cool for 10 minutes. Refrigerate, and serve chilled.

Rich Dark Chocolate Mousse

And now, for the piece de resistance! This is one of my favourite desserts, it's rich and creamy and full of anti-oxidant goodness. Add some fresh blueberries or strawberries, and you've got a winner that everyone will love.

Eating chocolate that is 70% cocoa content may seem intense and bitter at first, but you do get used to the flavour after a while. This is a great introduction to eating 70% chocolate, as the coconut milk and honey help to offset the decadent richness of the chocolate, while the addition of berries will give you a burst of fresh fruity flavour.

Ingredients:

3 tablespoons high fat cocoa powder

1/4 cup (40g) Arrowroot powder (also called Tapioca flour)

1 teaspoon vanilla extract

1 can (400ml) coconut milk

120g good-quality dark chocolate *(ideally with 70% cocoa content)*

2 tablespoons honey

2 large egg yolks, beaten

How To Make Rich Dark Chocolate Mousse

In a medium bowl, combine the cocoa powder, arrowroot powder and vanilla. Add about 2 or 3 tablespoons of the coconut milk, and whisk until it is smooth.

Bring the remaining coconut milk to a low simmer in a saucepan over medium heat. Break the chocolate into chunks and add it to the saucepan, stirring often, until melted.

Add the cocoa, arrowroot and vanilla mixture, continuously whisking.

Add a little bit of the warm chocolate mixture to the beaten egg yolks in a small bowl. Mix together well, and then add it all back into the saucepan and return to the heat.

Continue whisking the mixture until smooth, and it becomes thick enough to coat the back of a spoon.

Pour into small ramekins, and allow to cool for about 10 minutes. Place glad-wrap over the ramekins to prevent a skin forming on the chocolate, then put them in the fridge to cool down.

Serve cold, with fresh blueberries or strawberries on top.

Chapter 11
The Final Word

Modern lifestyle factors have placed a great deal of stress on our bodies, and the way we are genetically designed to function. When we talk about modern lifestyle factors, this really includes everything from the beginning of the Agricultural Revolution, 10,000 years ago, right up to now, as that was a relatively "modern" event in human history, and indeed, the history of the world.

The information I've shared with you here in this book may shock you at first, as a lot of it goes against the "conventional wisdom" that grains and dairy are good for us, that we need to eat lots of carbs, and that fat and cholesterol are all evil.

Scientific evidence based on millions of years of human history, eating habits, and anatomical discoveries, have led to the conclusions you find here in this book, and this has been backed up by scientists and nutritionists such as Dr Loren Cordain, Robb Wolf, Mark Sisson, and many other Paleo enthusiasts who have gone on to lose weight and gain energy simply by eating like our hunter-gatherer caveman ancestors.

I urge you to re-read the book if you have any remaining doubts, and to follow up with your own research as well if you wish.

There are many marketing giants around the world that have a vested interest in your eating habits, and therefore will only tell you part of the story about what you put into your mouth, and hoping your sugar addiction will continue lining their pockets. This list includes Big Pharma companies, who profit from all sorts of "magic pills" they offer the general public to solve their health problems.

I have no such agenda.

My only goal is to help you, your friends, and your family, to improve your health, lose weight, and gain energy. If I can just do that, then I'll consider myself successful.

The bottom line is, what you put in your body affects what your body does, and how you feel. If you focus on eating quality fresh organic produce, grass-fed meats, wild-caught seafood and healthy natural fats, then your body will respond by rewarding you with more energy to do the things you love to do, like play with your kids, or just to play in general.

By choosing quality food options similar to what Paleo man must have eaten 10,000 years ago, your body will become much more efficient at using the valuable nutrients you give it, and over time, all the excess baggage that has been built up will start to come off. By getting all of the quality nutrients you need from your diet, you will also reduce the chance of illness or disease, such as diabetes, heart disease, cancer, obesity, and many more.

Many of today's health problems can be solved by simply eating good quality food that our body needs to function at a high level.

Food is simply fuel for your body, to help you get through your busy day of activity. Hopefully I've also shown you that choosing quality fuel to provide your body doesn't necessarily mean the end of taste and flavour either.

Healthy and delicious food can all go together in the same sentence. The recipes I've provided here are a small sample of my favourite regular meals at home. Many of my friends wish I could cook for them every day!

I considered putting the meals together in the form of a 7 day plan, but I decided against it, as our ancestors never had that luxury.

So here's my simple guide for you...

If you feel like eating, then eat! Eat till you feel just satisfied, and then stop. Your body will tell you when it's had enough food, you just need to listen to the signals.

Eating plenty of protein and healthy fats will help to satiate your body and allow you to feel full for longer, so that in a couple of hours you aren't coming back for a snack.

Walk everywhere you can, and if you feel like going for a run, sprint! If you get up in the morning and you're feeling sore or you just can't be bothered doing much, then rest. There's no need to push yourself to exhaustion, it will just increase the stress on your body.

Make sure you lift something heavy every so often. Plyometric exercises and interval running are two of the best ways to increase your fitness, and both require short sharp bursts of high intensity, followed by a period of rest, so keep that in mind.

And most importantly, take time out to play and have some fun! Life is not meant to be so serious.

If you've found this book full of valuable information, and at least mildly entertaining, then I would urge you to share it with any loved ones you care about, including family, friends, and especially your children or grandchildren.

I hope that you start to take action for yourself, and also to lead the way and set a positive example for your children to follow, and their children, and so on.

You can find much more information to help you along your health and fitness path as well as lots of tasty new recipes to feed your inner caveman, at www.fitnessandhealthylifestyle.com.

Resources Section

aboutpaleodiet.org

altmed.creighton.edu

ehow.com

fitnessandhealthylifestyle.com

health.usnews.com

healthhabits.ca

hubpages.com

huffingtonpost.com

livestrong.com

livingpaleo.com

mattmetzgar.com

mendeley.com

ncbi.nlm.nih.gov

paleodietguru.com

paleodietlifestyle.com

paleodietnews.com

paleoforlife.org

paleovillage.com

pbs.org

scribd.com

webmd.com

The Paleo Solution by Robb Wolf

www.robbwolf.com

The Paleo Diet by Dr Loren Cordain

www.thepaleodiet.com

The Primal Blueprint by Mark Sisson

www.marksdailyapple.com

The Prehistoric World by Dougal Dixon

The Agile Gene by Matt Ridley

www.krispin.com

Paleo Comfort Foods by Julie and Charles Mayfield

The Primal Blueprint Cookbook by Mark Sisson with Jennifer Meier

Wikipedia.org